Olutoke Akande

Phone no 2348065741243

Email –akandereal@gmail.com

Medicinal Honey

Honey Healing Power

Olutoke Akande

INTRODUCTION

Many races especially Africa, Asia and Europe with America have used honey hundreds of years to nourish their body and cure ailments. Discover the secret of longer healthy life without illness in your life.

Honey cures and prevents all kinds of sickness of Skin, Teeth, Gums, Nails, Bones, Muscles, Lungs, Liver, Heart, Stomach, Intestine, Kidney, Vain, Nerves, Eyes, Nose, Throat, Ear, Hair, Bladder, Testes, Vagina, Womb, Babies, and lots more.

Benefits of raw Honey

- Honey is the food of the brain; it calms your blood pressure and makes you sleep well

- Honey helps medicines to cure you faster

- Honey clear your throat gives you fine voice

- Mood

- Honey wades off spiritual brain attack, increase your life spam more, refreshes your mind and keeps you younger and in good

- Honey keeps you intelligent and active

- Honey gives you good eyesight and mental alertness.

- Honey relaxes your brain, absolves tension and prevents your heart from breakdown as oil lubricate engine.

- Honey prevents feet swelling traveling or in long sitting position of the feet with exercise

- Honey cures stress, depression and bad dreams

- Honey immunizes you against sudden sickness by suppressing infections and diseases in the body

- Honey neutralizes toxic and poison in your body

HOW TO CURE MEASLES WITH HONEY

Ingredient

Honey

Bitter leave juice

Palm wine

How to prepare it

Add honey with bitter leaves juice and fresh palm wine .take a half cup daily and also rob on the skin

HOW TO CURE WATERY SPERM WITH HONEY

Ingredient

Honey

Mango root

How to prepare it

Add honey with fermented mango root. Take a half cup thrice daily. Eat food rich in protein. Abstain from sex a while. Avoid masturbation.

HOW TO CURE WEAK VAGINA WITH HONEY

Ingredient

Honey

Instruction

Take honey to relax your mind and exercise for muscles control in your pelvic. Try other sex variation.

HOW TO CURE TUBERCULOSIS WITH HONEY

Ingredient

Honey

Aloe Vera juice

Ginger

Garlic powder

Bitter kola,

Africa black pepper

How to prepare it

Add honey with aloe Vera juice, ginger, garlic powder, bitter kola, and African black pepper.

Dosage

Take two table spoons twice daily

HOW TO CURE AGING FACE WITH HONEY

Ingredient

Honey

Lime juice

Lotion or cream of your choice

How to prepare it and apply

Mix honey a little with cream or lotion and rob on face or mix honey with lime juice and rob on face daily. Wash face frequently.

Ingredient

Honey

Ointment

How to prepare it

Mix honey with ointment and massage. Stretch for the area and massage vigorously.

HOW TO CURE WHOOPING COUGH WITH HONEY

Ingredient

Honey

Native apple leaves

Lime

Garlic

How to prepare it

Mix honey with native apple leaves, lime and garlic, boiled with water and take one cup daily.

HOW TO CURE PRE- WHITE HAIRS WITH HONEY

How to prepare it

Rob a little honey on hairs overnight. Avoid shaving cream or too frequent use of it. Avoid stress. Avoid heat on hair. Avoid chemical on hair

HOW TO CURE BAD DREAMS WITH HONEY

Take little honey while going to bed. Avoid overeating before going to bed. Avoid horror movies before going to bed avoid stress and notice

HOW TO CURE LIPS SORE WITH HONEY

Ingredient

Honey

Vitamin c tablet

How to prepare it

 Take table spoon of honey daily. With vitamin C tablets. Treat malaria. Keep sore dry and hygienic.

HOW TO CURE BODY HEAT WITH HONEY

Take honey twice daily. Treat malaria stay in a well ventilated area. Frequent cold bath.

HOW TO CURE BABY RASHES WITH HONEY

Ingredient

Honey

Sheer butter

Red canniual flower

Lime juice

How to prepare it

Mix a little honey with a mixture of sheer butter, red canniual flower and lime juice bulbs bath and rob the baby's skin

HOW TO CURE OVERNIGHT PAINS WITH HONEY

Ingredient

Honey

Paracetamol

Anti – rheumatism medicine

How to prepare and apply it

Take 3 table spoon of honey with paracetamol and anti – rheumatism medicine. Avoid lying on hard surface overnight.

HOW TO CURE HOT BREATH WITH HONEY

Ingredient

Milk

Honey

How to prepare it

Take a cup of milk mixed with honey. Treat malarial fever

HOW TO CURE MOUTH ODOUR WITH HONEY

Dip toothpaste in honey and brush. Rinse mouth with water after meal, juice or alcohol. Wash your tongue once in two weeks.

HOW TO CURE JOINT PAIN WITH HONEY

Ingredient

Honey

Neem (azadirachta indica) leaves juice

How to prepare it

Mix honey with boil neem leaves juice and takes one cup daily. Take any body pain of your choice and anti-rheumatism tablets. Avoid overwork or exercise.

HOW TO CURE STRAIN VEINS WITH HONEY

Massage the part with honey and ointment. Stretch forth to and fro. Take pain relieve tablets. Exercise.

HOW TO CURE INFLAMED NOSE

Press nose with hot towel. Rob nose with honey mixed with lime juice. Rob nose with sulphur

HOW TO CURE CHILD SLOW GROWTH WITH HONEY

Ingredient

Honey

Aloe Vera juice

How to prepare it

Mix honey with aloe Vera juice and add into the child's meal. Eat food rich in proteins like milk, egg, beans and soya beans.

HOW TO CURE SWOLLEN EYES WITH HONEY

Ingredient

Honey

Milk

How to prepare it

Add honey with milk in a cup and take before going to bed. Enough sleep and rest. Drink enough water. Avoid alcohol. Eat well with Fruits and vegetable.

HOW TO CURE OILY NOSE WITH HONEY

Squeeze nose and wash with a solution of lime juice and honey. Good face hygiene. Press nose with hot towel one daily.

HOW TO CURE BAD CATARACT WITH HONEY

Put two drops of clean honey into the eyes two time daily

HOW TO CURE BIG TUMMY WITH HONEY

Take honey after, exercise, exercise the tummy. Avoid alcohol that can cause inflammation of your internal organs. Reduce intake of oil and fat food.

HOW TO CURE TRAVEL SWOLLEN FEET WITH HONEY

Ingredient

Honey

Water

How to prepare it

Add honey in a half cup of water and take before traveling.
Drink water at intervals. Feet stretching at intervals.
Regular walking exercise. Eat fruits.

HOW TO CURE RUNNING NOSE WITH HONEY

Ingredient

Honey

Lime juice

How to prepare it

Mix 6 table spoon of honey with lime juice and take twice
daily. Observe siesta and rest. Stay in a ventilated area.
Use relief ointment

HOW TO CURE OVERNIGHT STIFF NECK WITH HONEY

Ingredient

Honey

Paracetamol or any pain relieve tablet

Anti- rheumatism

How to prepare it

Exercise your neck. Take a glass of warm water mixed with 4 table spoon of honey. Take paracetamol or any pain relieve tablet and anti rheumatism tablet. Correct sleeping position

HOW TO CURE PIN PIES ACNE WITH HONEY

Ingredient

Honey

Lime juice

How to prepare and apply it

Mix a half table spoon of honey with lime juice and rob on face twice daily. Press face with hot towel. Apply suphur. Good face hygiene.

HOW TO CURE NOSE BLEEDING WITH HONEY

Ingredient

Honey

Scent leaves juice

How to prepare it

Mix honeys with scent leaves juice and apply. Do not press nose stop blood. Avoid direct sun and long trekking in the sun

HOW TO CURE BLACK SPOTS WITH HONEY

Ingredient

Honey

Lime juice

How to prepare it

Add honey with lime juice and rob face. Use non bleaching medicated soap use specialize lotion

HOW TO CURE ECZEMA WITH HONEY

Ingredient

Honey

Lime juice

Sulphur creams

How to prepare and apply it

Mix honey with lime juice and sulphur creams. Rob the area. Bath with medicated soap. Don't share cloths and towel with vitamins.

HOW TO CURE BODY BRUISES WITH HONEY

Ingredient

Honey

Ointment

How to prepare and apply it

Add drop of honey into ointment and apply. Wash area with disinfectant. Keep dry and clean. Take body pain tables.

HOW TO CURE SWEATING ARMPIT WITH HONEY

Scrap hairs regularly with a shaving blade. Apply honey and wash. Take bath frequently. Wash armpit before work.

HOW TO CURE SNORING WITH HONEY

Take 3 table spoon of honey before sleep. Sleep on soft Material. Sleep in good ventilated area. Avoid alcohol and over eating before sleep. Avoid eating lying to sleep.

HOW TO CURE BODY RASHES WITH HONEY

Ingredient

Honey

Ointment

Anti- rashes cream

How to prepare it

Rob honey on the patches 2 times daily use anti – rashes specialize cream or ointment. Avoid scratching to become wound.

HOW TO CURE WATER EXCREMENT WITH HONEY

Ingredient

Honey

Sweet basil leaves

Aloe Vera

How to prepare it

Mix honey with sweet basil leaves and aloe Vera and take 4 times daily. Avoid eating between meals. Avoid long hunger and spoilt food.

Ingredient

Honey

Aloe Vera juice

How to apply it

Mix honey with aloe Vera juice. Apply after bath twice daily. Rob petroleum jelly or paraffin oil on skin.

HOW TO CURE HEART/CHEST PAIN WITH HONEY

Blend together honey, onion and garlic. Take I table spoon twice daily.

HOW TO CURE INFECTED WOUND WITH HONEY

Ingredient

Honey

Fresh pawpaw stem juice

How to apply it

Mix drop of honey on fresh pawpaw stem juice. Apply on the wound. Keep wound dry and net

Make a tea infusion of mistle toe and sweeten it with honey. Take a half glass twice daily.

HOW TO CURE BOIL WITH HONEY

Ingredient

Honey

Ointment

Garlic

Sheer butter

How to prepare it

Mix honey with sheer butter, garlic and apply on boil. Keep boil free from dirt and fire. Apply boil specialize ointment. Take body pain tablet of your choice.

HOW TO CURE DANDRUFF WITH HONEY

Ingredient

Honey

Anti dandruff cream

How to apply it

Mix little honey with anti dandruff cream and apply on head after skin cut. Wash lead with medicated soap regularly.

HOW TO CURE EXCESS MENSES WITH HONEY

Ingredient

Honey

Cotton pods

Refers to menstruation exceeding the normal period. Honey with boiled cotton pods. Add water and take 1 glass twice daily.

HOW TO CURE EAR ITCHING WITH HONEY

Ingredient

Honey

Little salt

Warm water

How to prepare it

Mix honey with a little salt and warm water and apply two drops before bet time. Clean ear with wool. Once in every two weeks.

HOW TO CURE SWOLLEN GUMS WITH HONEY

Ingredient

Honey

Aloe Vera juice

Tooth paste

How to prepare it

Make a paste of aloe Vera juice and tooth paste, add honey and vitamin C powder, apply on the tooth mouth one daily. Don't brush your gums. Keep mouth hygienic

HOW TO CURE INSECT STING WITH HONEY

Ingredient

Aloe Vera leave

Sheer butter

Lime juice

Honey

How to prepare it

Blend aloe Vera leaves, sheer butter, lime juice and honey. Apply the paste on the area. Apply anti insect venom cream. Take any body pain tablet.

HOW TO CURE WAIST PAIN WITH HONEY

Ingredient

Honey

Anti rheumatism

And body pain of your choice

How to prepare it

Take honey before bedtime. Avoid overwork. Good rest and sleep. Take anti rheumatism and anybody pain tablet of your choice.

HOW TO CURE BLADDER INFECTION WITH HONEY

Ingredient

Cinnamon powder

Honey

How to prepare it

Mix two table spoon of cinnamon powder with a half table spoon of honey in a half cup of warm water and take once daily

HOW TO CURE EYE TWINKLING WITH HONEY

Ingredient

Milk

Honey

Multivitamin

How to prepare it

Drink a cup of warm water, mixed with honey and milk daily. Take multivitamin and mineral capsule. Drink enough water daily

HOW TO CURE STAIN TEETH WITH HONEY

Brush teeth with honey and little toothpaste before going to sleep. Brush teeth twice daily. Rinse mouth after meal; avoid drinking alcohol and eating kola nut.

HOW TO CURE BLEEDING WOUND WITH HONEY

Apply honey mixed with fresh banana fluid on the wound. Keep wound clean.

HOW TO CURE BACK PAIN WITH HONEY

Take honey before going to bed. Don't over work yourself in one bending position for long. Enough rest and sleep. Take anti rheumatism and paracetamol tablet.

HOW TO CURE NOISY BOWELS WITH HONEY

Ingredient

Honey

Lemon juice

Milk

How to prepare it

Mix honey with lemon juice and milk in a glass of warm water and take. Drink water at intervals. Avoid overeating between meals or going to bed. Avoid hunger

HOW TO CURE EYE ITCHING WITH HONEY

Ingredient

Aloe Vera juice

Honey

How to prepare it

Make an eyes drop of honey and aloe Vera juice, mix and put two drops on the eye twice daily. Take yeast tablet or fresh palm wine.

HOW TO CURE WATERY EYES WITH HONEY

Wash eyes thoroughly with ordinary water make an eye drop of honey and aloe Vera, drop two daily. Keep eyes away from air/ chemical pollution

Ingredient

Aloe Vera

Honey

Avocado peer

How to prepare it

Mix honey with aloe Vera juice and the paste of avocado peer, rob on your skin after bath before going to bed. Bath with medicated soap, use cream/lotion rich in vitamin E.A

HOW TO CURE WRINKLES WITH HONEY

Mix little honey with your cream or lotion and rob. Use specialize cream. Do not squeeze your face out of habit. Observe your siesta.

HOW TO CURE TOOTH PAIN WITH HONEY

Ingredient

Honey

Cinnamon powder

How to prepare it

Mix 2-3 table spoon of honey with paste of one table spoon of cinnamon powder

Dosage

Apply on the aching tooth 2 times after meal. Take calcium and vitamin c tables daily use fluoride rich tooth paste.

HOW TO CURE WEEK ERECTION WITH HONEY

Ingredient

Honey

Onion juice

Boiled egg

Fiber food

Water

How to prepare it

Mix 3 table spoon of honey with cooked onion juice.

Dosage

Take 2 times daily, eat half boiled egg eat food rich in fibre. Drink plenty of water. Avoid much sugar and alcohol rest and sleep well

HOW TO CURE DRY AND WRINKLE SKIN WITH HONEY

Ingredient

Honey

Any cream or lotion

How to prepare it

Mix a little honey with your cream or lotion and use cream or lotion rich in vitamin A and E. apply paraffin oil on your skin

HOW TO CURE HAIR LOSS WITH HONEY

Ingredient

Honey

Olive oil

How to prepare it

Mix honey with warm olive oil, apply on hairs before wash weekly. Avoid frequent perming of hairs and chemicals stop using fake chemical or relaxers on hairs

HOW TO CURE COLD AND COUGH WITH HONEY

Ingredient

Honey

Garlic

Lemon juice

How to prepare it

Mix honey with glove of garlic soaked in lemon juice

Dosage

Drink the mixture. Use anti cold and cough medicines.
Protect yourself against infected persons.

Other Books

1. Medicinal Honey and Healing Properties

2. Medicinal Honey: HONEY HEALING POWER

3. 14 New Ways to Stop Masturbation

4. More than 200 Sicknesses Honey can cure

5. Prophetic Dreaming

6. Loss weight in less than three weeks with Homemade Drink

7. Prayer: Prayer that force God into Action

8. The strategy

They are available in Amazon kindle book

Click here to leave a review for this book on Amazon

Thank you and good luck

URL

http://www.amazon.com/author/olutokeakande

http://www.amazon.com/author/john123